Idrissa Sacko

Health and Safety at Work and Professional Environments in Mali

Idrissa Sacko

Health and Safety at Work and Professional Environments in Mali

ScienciaScripts

Imprint

Any brand names and product names mentioned in this book are subject to trademark, brand or patent protection and are trademarks or registered trademarks of their respective holders. The use of brand names, product names, common names, trade names, product descriptions etc. even without a particular marking in this work is in no way to be construed to mean that such names may be regarded as unrestricted in respect of trademark and brand protection legislation and could thus be used by anyone.

Cover image: www.ingimage.com

This book is a translation from the original published under ISBN 978-620-3-44503-9.

Publisher:
Sciencia Scripts
is a trademark of
Dodo Books Indian Ocean Ltd. and OmniScriptum S.R.L publishing group

120 High Road, East Finchley, London, N2 9ED, United Kingdom
Str. Armeneasca 28/1, office 1, Chisinau MD-2012, Republic of Moldova, Europe
Printed at: see last page
ISBN: 978-620-8-04736-8

ASSESSMENT OF PHYSICAL AND CHEMICAL HAZARDS IN ORTHOPEDIC APPLIANCE MANUFACTURING WORKSHOPS AT THE MALI NATIONAL ORTHOPEDIC APPLIANCE CENTER

I Sacko[1] , TB Bagayoko[2] , (SOMASST)[3]

1. Mali National Orthopedic Fitting Center
2. Forensic and occupational medicine department at the Nianankoro Fomba hospital in Ségou.
3. Société Malienne de Santé Sécurité au Travail

Author: Dr Idrissa Sacko, Occupational Health and Safety Specialist, Centre National d'Appareillage Orthopédique. 00223 76 18 88 82

Email : sackoidrissa43@yahoo.fr

Conflict of interest: none.

Summary: In Mali, the Centre National d'Appareillage Orthopédique du Mali (CNAOM) provides specialized orthopedic and rehabilitation services. It also specializes in the design and promotion of appliances and technical aids for disabled people.

Objective: Evaluate physical and chemical hazards in orthopedic appliance manufacturing workshops.

Methodology: This was a descriptive cross-sectional study from August 1 to 31, 2020. All orthoprosthetists working in production workshops were included. Technical visits to the premises and a multi-part questionnaire (socio-demographic aspects, working conditions, etc.) were carried out. Data were collected in production areas for environmental metrology (noise, ambient temperature, dust, light).

Results: There was a clear male predominance, with a sex ratio of 6.5% in favour of men. The average age was 40.25 years, with extremes of 20 and 60 years. Length of service of less than 5 years was 60.0% among workers. Over half the workers were orthoprosthetists. In the machine room, metrology revealed a noise level of 90 dB(A), discomfort in the heat, with temperatures ranging from 26 to 40°C, and the amount of light provided did not meet standards. The amount of plaster dust found in the ambient air was 5.5 mg/cm3 in the plastering and molding room. We noted the presence of numerous chemicals in the working environment. In terms of occupational accidents encountered by workers, 53.3% found they were more exposed to injuries, 13.3% found they were exposed to cuts, 73.3% to burns. In terms of personal protective equipment, 86.6% wore masks. As for the use of gloves, only 66.6% had them and used them from time to time. We did not record any cases of occupational illness.

Conclusion: Prosthesis manufacturing activities expose workers to numerous risks, with the simultaneous presence of several hazardous work situations. Hence the need to consider prevention strategies focusing primarily on primary prevention.

<u>Key words</u>: assessment; physical and chemical nuisances; orthopedic appliances; workshops; CNAOM.

INTRODUCTION

In Mali, the Centre National d'Appareillage Orthopédique du Mali (CNAOM) provides specialized orthopedic and rehabilitation services. It also specializes in the design and promotion of appliances and technical aids for disabled people;
A prosthesis is a device used to replace an amputated limb, part of a limb or a severely damaged or destroyed organ. [1]

In the workplace, workers may be exposed simultaneously to numerous chemical and physical agents. The multiplicity and concomitance of these exposures can favor the onset of pathologies and accentuate the arduousness of work. [2].

To make a prosthesis, we start with the mold, which is used to measure the amputated part. This measurement gives the negative (the magnon imprint), from which we obtain the positive (mold). Once the positive has been obtained, it undergoes thermoforming, and the equipment for any prosthesis is assembled. In the fitting room, the patient begins to walk.

The different types of prostheses are :

- Tibial prosthesis: a device used to replace part of the foot amputated at the femur;
- Femoral prosthesis: a device used to replace the femur amputated above;

- Upper limb prosthesis: a device used to replace an amputated upper limb [10].

During these stages, many of the products used are recognized as toxic, such as acetone, neoprene glue, resin and metals. Some of these agents are responsible for sometimes serious conditions such as cancer, asthma and silicosis, which remains the most frequently described occupational disease among dental technicians. It is linked to the inhalation of siliceous dust during the manufacture of molds for metal prostheses. Denture manufacture also requires the use of machines and ovens, which can cause noise pollution, heatstroke and burns [1].

In view of the absence of such a study at CNAOM and the difficult professional context of health and safety risks for workers, we initiated this study. We decided to focus solely on assessing the physical and chemical hazards to which workers are exposed.

I-MATERIALS AND METHOD

1.1- Study setting: The study was carried out at the Centre National d'Appareillage Orthopédique du Mali (CNAOM).

1.2- Type and period of study: This was a descriptive cross-sectional study from August 1 to 31, 2020.

1.3- Study population: The study concerned orthoprosthetists working in the manufacturing workshops of the Centre National d'Appareillage Orthopédique du Mali and the prosthesis production areas.

1.4- Sampling: All orthoprosthetists were included in the study. Workshops and workstations were also included in the samples for ambient measurements.

1.5- Inclusion criteria: All exposed orthoprosthetists and their workstations were included in our study.

1.6- Non-inclusion criteria: Any person who did not wish to answer the questionnaire was excluded from the study.

1.7- Data collection techniques and tools: An individual, anonymous questionnaire was administered to each employee. In addition to socio-demographic and occupational data, the questionnaire included measurements of nuisances in the work environment. The data collected were processed using SPSS (version 20.0) and EXCEL (version 17) software, and the text was processed using Microsoft Word.

<u>**II- RESULT**</u>

1- Socio-demographic characteristics of participants

<u>**Table I:**</u> Age distribution.

Age	Workforce	Percentage
20 to 30 years	3	20
31 to 40 years	9	60
41 to 50 years	2	13,7
51 to 60 years	1	6,7
Total	15	100,0

Table II: Breakdown by gender.

Gender	Workforce	Percentage
Men	13	86,7
Woman	2	13,3
Total	15	100,0

Table III: Breakdown by qualification.

Qualification	Workforce	Percentage
Orthoprosthetist	8	53,3
Orthoprosthetist's Helper	7	46,7
Total	15	100,0

Table IV: Breakdown by seniority.

Seniority	Workforce	Percentage
Under5years	9	60,0
5 to 10 years	2	13,3
10 to 15 years	1	6,7
Plus15years	3	20,0
Total	15	100,0

Figure1: Plaster for prostheses.

Figure2: Prosthesis: tibial, femoral, crutch.

<u>**III- DISCUSSION**</u>

With a mean age of 40.25 years and extremes of 20 and 60 years, our result is lower than that of I.N.A AKA et al [1]. And higher than that of Benzarti Mezni, A. et al [3] who found an average age of 37.1 years. We noted a clear male predominance, with a sex ratio of 6.5% in favor of men. Our result is comparable to that of Amel Arib et al (Mezdad, Mohamed, & Mohamed, 2016) [4]. This could be explained by the fact that women consider this profession to be simply for men. Seniority at less than 5 years was 60.0% among workers, our result is lower than that of S AD et al [5]. . In the machine room, metrology revealed a noise level of 90 dB(A), discomfort in the heat, with temperatures ranging from 26 to 40°C, and the amount of light provided did not meet standards. The amount of plaster dust found in the ambient air was 5.5 mg/cm3 in the plastering and molding room. We noted the presence of numerous chemicals in the working environment. Noise annoyance is a difficult concept to quantify: everyone is well aware of the difference in appreciation of a noise and a musical atmosphere of equal sound level, for example, or according to the time of day when it occurs, its duration, or the ambient noise level. Noise can become annoying when, because of its nature, frequency or intensity, it is likely to cause excessive disturbance to people, danger, harm to health or damage to the environment [6]. In a study carried out in Côte d'Ivoire by B Y Yeboué et al [7], noise exposure in excess of 90 dB(A) for more than 2 hours was found to be more frequent in the timber industry and secondarily in agro-industry, and similar to that of a study carried out in Burkina Faso by O Souleymane et al [8]. N'Diaye et al. in Senegal (N'Diaye et al. 2014) found an exposure duration of 16 to 30 years [9].in Mali a study by Bagayoko TB et al found values oscillating between 70 and 105 dB for 82% at workstation levels [11]. The noise came from the machine room. They were exposed to it discontinuously and at medium intensity. In terms of work-related accidents, 53.3% of workers were more exposed to injuries, 13.3% to cuts and 73.3% to burns. As means of protection, 100% had work clothes. We found that this work clothing was not very adequate. As for other means of personal protection, 86.6% wore masks. As for the use of gloves, only 66.6% had them and used them from time to time. We did not record any cases of occupational illness.

<u>**IV- BIBLIOGRAPHICAL REFERENCES**</u>

[1] **I.NA. AKA et al:** Assessment of physical and chemical nuisances in an orthopedic appliance manufacturing workshop at the Yopougon-Abidjan University Hospital.

 https://www.sciencedirect.com/journal/archives-des-maladies-professionnelles-et-de-lenvironnement/vol/77/issue/4   September 2016, Pages 665-669

[2] **Nadine Fréry et al:** EXPOSURE OF EMPLOYEES TO MULTIPLE CARCINOGENIC NUISANCES IN 2010. Soumis le 10.03.2017 // Date of submission: 03.10.2017

[3] **Benzarti Mezni, A. et al**. (2014). "Profil Étiologique Des Surdités d'origine Professionnelle. À Propos de 67 Cas." Archives des Maladies Professionnelles et de l'Environnement 75(3): S21. **https://linkinghub.elsevier.com/retrieve/pii/S1775878514001076.**

[4] **Mezdad Amel Arib Ep, Amer Lamara Mahamed, & Amer Lamara Mahamed (2016):** Évaluation Du Déficit Auditif Moyen Chez Les Travailleurs D'Une Industrie De L'Électroménager." Archives des Maladies Professionnelles et de l'Environnement 77(3): 539. **https://linkinghub.elsevier.com/retrieve/pii/S177587851630460X.**

[5] **S A DIA et al**: Assessment of occupational risks in the artisanal aluminum foundry sector in Dakar.

https://www.sciencedirect.com/journal/archives-des-maladies-professionnelles-et-de-lenvironnement. October 2017, Pages 454-459

[6] MATCHUM KOUOGUE CHRISTELLE F.-A.: La protection juridique de l'environnement au Cameroun et en France le cas des nuisances sonores. University of Limoges - Master 2 thesis in International and Comparative Environmental Law 2008.

[7] B Y Yeboué et al: Assessment of noise risk at 881 workstations in 320 private sector companies in Côte d'Ivoire. https://www.sciencedirect.com/journal/archives-des-maladies-professionnelles-et-de-lenvironnement/vol/79/issue/4. September 2018, Pages 528-533

[8] O Souleymane et al: Impact des Nuisances Sonores sur la Qualité de Vie des Travailleurs dans les Centrales Électriques de la Ville de Ouagadougou. European Scientific Journal March 2019 edition Vol.15, No.9 ISSN: 1857 - 7881 (Print) e - ISSN 1857- 7431

[9] N'Diaye, M. et al (2014): "Évaluation Du Risque Bruit Au Niveau Du

Site Acide Des Industries Chimiques Du Sénégal (ICS)." Archives des Maladies Professionnelles et de l'Environnement 75(3): S19. https://linkinghub.elsevier.com/retrieve/pii/S1775878514001015.

[10] : Unité des Études, Recherche, Documentation et Informatique CNAOM ; Ordonnance N°2-065 du 18 décembre 2002 portant création du CNAOM

[11] **Bagayoko TB et al :** Evaluation des facteurs d'ambiances physiques de travail à la Compagnie Malienne de Textile (COMATEX-SA), SEGOU. MALI SANTE PUBLIQUE, December 2020 TOME X N° 02

ASSESSMENT OF OCCUPATIONAL RISKS IN A MODERN CAR GARAGE IN BAMAKO

I Sacko[1] , TB Bagayoko[2] , Z Coulibaly[3] , M Diawara[4] , S Sanogo[5,] B Diallo[6] , L Diakité[7] , FB TOURE[8] , B GAKOU[9] , P Hamidou[10,] (SOMASST) [11]

4. National Orthopedic Fitting Center of Mali

5. Forensic and occupational medicine department at the Nianankoro Fomba hospital in Ségou.

6. Institut National de Prévoyance Sociale (Mali)

7. Caisse Nationale d'Assurance Mali (Mali)

8. Agence Nationale d'Assistance Médicale (Bamako Mali)

9. Caisse Malienne de Sécurité Sociale (Mali)

10. Pelengana Sud Community Health Center (Ségou Mali)

11. Institut National de Prévoyance Sociale (Mali)

12. Cabinet Médical KENEYA (Bamako Mali)

13. Caisse Malienne de Sécurité Sociale (Mali)

14. Société Malienne de Santé Sécurité au Travail.

Author: Dr Idrissa Sacko, Occupational Health and Safety Specialist, National Orthopedic Fitting Center. 00223 76 18 88 82 Email : sackoidrissa43@yahoo.fr

Summary: Occupational risks, as represented by work-related accidents and illnesses, are the cause of significant personal injury, material damage, financial losses and a deterioration in the social climate within companies.

Aim: the aim of our study was to assess occupational hazards in a modern car garage in the city of Bamako.

Methodology: This was a descriptive cross-sectional study conducted over a two-month period. All garage staff, regardless of age or qualifications, were included. Data were collected through site visits and a multi-part questionnaire (socio-demographic aspects, working conditions and risk assessment).

Results: The mean age **was** 30 years, and exclusively male. The extremes were 19 and 54 years. Half the garage staff had more than 10 years' seniority. Monthly income was low. The main activity was breakdown service, bodywork, painting and rapid maintenance. Within the garage, among the nuisance factors we recorded, 50% were exposed to heat and dust, 75% to noise, 50% to fumes and steam, and 65% to vibrations. The risk of explosion or fire was 80%. No cases of occupational deafness were recorded. With regard to constraints linked to work situations, all (100%) claimed to adopt different postures in practice, some more uncomfortable than others. 90% of these workers did more handling. Mental workload was also very high, with 50% claiming to have it. 85% had had 1 to 2 work-related accidents, while 15% claimed to have had between 3 and 4, and 20% reported a commuting accident. **Conclusion:** The car garage is a high-risk workplace, with the simultaneous presence of several hazards and dangerous work situations. In this environment, it is important to consider prevention strategies focusing primarily on primary prevention.

<u>Key words</u>: assessment; occupational hazards; garage, Bamako

INTRODUCTION

Occupational risks, as represented by workplace accidents and occupational illnesses, are the cause of significant personal injury, material damage, financial losses and a deterioration in the social climate within companies.

In 2005, the frequency of workplace accidents was 5 to 7 times higher in (very) small companies with fewer than 20 employees than in establishments with 1,500 or more employees. There are a number of reasons for these results, which are all the more worrying given that the future of employment is often linked to the supposed dynamism of SMEs: more than elsewhere, risk is perceived as a component of the identity of the profession, while awareness of danger is dependent on direct confrontation with a serious accident, whereas in its absence, the status quo seems justifiable; responsibility is frequently blamed on individual behaviour and attitudes; the cost of accidents and work stoppages is largely underestimated [1]. Professional car repairers (mechanics, body repairers) are particularly exposed to carcinogenic, chemical and physical hazards in garage workshops and paint booths. The multiplicity and concomitance of these exposures can favour the onset of pathologies and accentuate hardship at work, as shown by the Health and Professional Itinerary survey carried out by the Direction de la recherche des études, de l'évaluation et des statistiques (Drees) and the Direction de l'animation de la recherche, des études et des statistiques (Dares) (SIP 2006-2010 1) [2]. Even today, a large number of accidents at work and occupational illnesses (AT/MP) occur in France during the course of work.

Every day, 170 workplace accidents result in permanent disability or death, and around 80 people are diagnosed with an occupational disease. This is not the only reason why risk assessment is necessary. The absence of an accident or occupational disease does not mean the absence of an accident or occupational disease.

that there is no risk: zero occupational injuries is not the same as zero risk.

Indeed, occupational risk assessment presupposes a proactive approach within the company, in order to understand and analyze all phenomena likely to give rise to a risk to health and safety in the workplace [3].

A priori risk assessment is an essential means of safeguarding staff health and safety, as part of an overall approach to preventing occupational hazards in higher education and research establishments [4]. Before delving into the bibliography on risk assessment, we thought it would be useful to define certain concepts [5].

Hazard (or dangerous phenomenon): a cause capable of causing injury or damage to health.

Hazardous situation: any situation in which a person is exposed to one or more hazards.

Hazardous event: event likely to cause damage to health.

Risk: combination of probability and severity of injury or damage to health that may occur in a hazardous situation [6].

Risk analysis: study of the conditions under which workers are exposed to these hazards

Risk assessment is defined as the appraisal of risks to workers' health and safety, in all work-related aspects (including organization, pace and duration of work) [7].

- The frequency of work-related accidents in the automotive repair sector in France,

- Lack of information for workers on the various risk factors and corrective and preventive measures in this environment,

- How to change the behavior of these workers

Our choice of theme.

I-MATERIALS AND METHOD

A- Type of study: This was a descriptive cross-sectional study.

B- Study period: The study took place over a 02-month period from October 1er 2014 to November 30 2014.

C- Study population: The study involved garage staff of all ages and qualifications.

D- Sampling :

1- Inclusion criteria: All personnel working in this garage during the study period.

2- Non-inclusion criteria: Administrative staff were excluded from the study.

E- Data collection tool: To carry out this survey, we developed a data collection form based on other forms used in other studies and on bibliographical research.

Developing the questionnaire was the most difficult stage of our research. We drew up two survey forms: one providing us with information on the company itself and the various risks to which workers are exposed, and the other on the employee and his or her work environment.

The company questionnaire includes questions divided into the following categories:

- Company identification,
- Work organization,
- Internal company risks,
- Equipment risks,
- The most commonly used postures,
- Means of protection available to employees,
- Recorded occupational illnesses and accidents.

- The employee questionnaire includes 06 categories of questions: semi-open and closed-ended. The form includes questions divided into the following categories:
- Employee identification,
- Activity,
- Risk assessment
- Means of protection,
- Work-related accidents,
- Occupational illnesses.

F- Data supports: The information gathered was available from :

- Gathering information by interview,

- Observation of work situations,

- Consultation of company documents relating to occupational categories, work sections, medical registers and the medical file of each worker,

- A company visit sheet for assessing occupational risks.

- The results of environmental measurements carried out at workstations by our team.

The measuring instruments used are :

- For noise : PYLE PSP01 sound level meter
- For temperature: TROTEC BP20 infrared thermometer
- For light intensity: TROTEC BF05 lux meter
- TROTEC BZ25 C02 Thermo-hygro-gasometer

G- Collection technique: We read the above-mentioned documents and recorded them on a questionnaire.

H- Data processing: Data were entered and analyzed using SPSS 12.0 software. Word processing was performed on Microsoft Word.

<u>**II- INCOME**</u>

<u>**Table I**</u>: Age distribution.

Age	Workforce	Percentage
19-24years	01	5
25-30 years	01	5
31-36 years old	03	15
37-42years	08	40
43-48years	04	20
49-54 years	03	15
TOTAL	20	100

<u>**Table II**</u>: Breakdown by gender.

Gender	Workforce	Percentage
MALE	20	100
FEMALE	00	00
TOTAL	20	100

<u>**Figure 1**</u>: Breakdown by seniority.

<u>**Table III**</u>: Breakdown by activity

Activity	Workforce	Percentage
Paint	05	25
Body shop	05	25
Troubleshooting	07	35
Fast maintenance	03	15
TOTAL	20	100

<u>**Figure 2:**</u> Distribution of workers according to nuisance factors

<u>**Table IV**</u>: Distribution of workers according to equipment-related risks

Equipment risks	Workforce	Percentage
CUT-OUT	05	25
INJURIES	18	90
ECRASEMENT	05	25
BURNS	05	25
TRAUMATISM	01	05

<u>**Figure3**</u>: Distribution of workers according to accident risk

<u>**III- DISCUSSION**</u>

This company's activities include: car sales, spare parts sales, car mechanics. It is a modern company. It has a workforce of 100 and is a member of the occupational health system, with an infirmary. The company's facilities include changing rooms, a catering system and toilets that comply with the relevant standards. The various risks in the garage vary according to the workstation. There are, however, a number of in-house risks to which they are all exposed: noise, heat, vibrations, lighting, fumes and dust. Equipment-related risks: cuts, injuries, crushing, burns, serious trauma, fire or explosion. The different postures used by all are :

- Standing, trunk in anteflexion and rotation,
- Crouching or kneeling,
- Supported by elbows or wrists,
- Arms in the air,
- Lying down, arms in the air,
- Leaning forward.

The garage provides employees with protective gear, and all workers are equipped with work clothes. There are registers in which accidents and occupational diseases are recorded. There have been a few cases of accidents which have been covered by the employer and the fund (Institut National de Prévoyance Sociale).

The average age **was** 30, and the patients were exclusively male. With extremes of 19 and 54, our result is lower than that of S A DIA et al [8], who found an average age of 40 and exclusively men. This could be explained by the fact that women consider this profession to be simply for men. Half the garage staff had a seniority of over 10 years, our result is higher than that of S AD et al [9]. Within the garage, among the nuisance factors we recorded, 50% of workers were bothered by heat, 50% by dust, 75% by noise, 50% by fumes and steam and 65% by vibrations. Noise annoyance is a difficult concept to quantify: everyone is well aware of the difference in appreciation of a noise and a musical atmosphere of equal sound level, for example, or according to the time of day when it occurs, its duration, or the ambient noise level. Noise can become a nuisance when, because of its nature, frequency or intensity, it is likely to cause excessive disturbance to people, danger, harm to health or damage to the environment [10]. Among nuisance factors, noise accounted for 75% of cases. Our result is lower than that of a study carried out in Côte d'Ivoire by B Y Yeboué et al [11], which found 98%. Noise was mainly due to motors, fittings, air compressor, impact wrench, extractors and pneumatic chisel. They were exposed to noise throughout the working day, but discontinuously and at moderate intensity. No cases of deafness were recorded. Mental workload was also very high, with 50% claiming to have it. With regard to constraints linked to work situations, all (100%) claimed to adopt different postures in practice, some more uncomfortable than others. In our study, 90% of these workers were involved in material handling. Mental workload was also very high, with 50% claiming to have it. This mental load can be explained by the pressure to which they are subjected by customers who want their vehicles back as soon as possible; and family needs. The human factor and the time factor play against them, which could lead to stress. Psychosocial risks concern work situations at risk of stress, internal violence and external violence. These risks may be induced by the activity itself or generated by the organization of work [12]. With regard to risks related to work equipment, workers found that they were more exposed to injuries in 90% of cases; given their versatility at the workstation, the lack of PPE worn and their lack of qualifications, they are therefore very frequently the victims of accidents at work without any major severity. The risk of falling consisted of falls on the same level on a slippery floor with dirty oil, a regular floor and a floor often strewn with obstacles. The risk of explosion or fire was 80%. This could be explained by the gas cylinder, which was poorly stored, and the many flammable products, including hydrocarbons, often found on the floor. Then there was the heat source (engines, exhausts, electricity and high temperatures). 85% had had 1 to 2 work-related accidents, while 15% claimed to have had between 3 and 4, and 20% reported a commuting accident. The various accidents ranged from simple cuts (15%) to injuries (60%). We did not record any cases of crushing.

CATHEL KORNIG AND ÉRIC VERDIER [3] found that 41% of accidents at work are linked to manual handling, 16% to accidents on the same level, 8% to falls from height, and 13% to tool falls, to name only the most frequent. These accidents cause, in order of frequency, wounds, contusions, lumbago, sprains or fractures. Mechanics are among the professions particularly exposed to the risk of low-back pain. The stakes of prevention are therefore high in a sector whose employers often complain of recruitment difficulties [13].Only 10% claimed to have had an occupational illness. 40% found they had muscular disorders and 50% skeletal disorders. These risks can also affect physical health (cardiovascular disease, musculoskeletal disorders, etc.) or mental health [14].

IV- BIBLIOGRAPHICAL REFERENCES

[1] ERIC VERDIER: PME et prévention des risques professionnels : difficile dialogue ou impossible rencontre? APRES-DEMAIN N12 01/10/09 Page34.
LA SANTÉ PUBLIQUE N° 12 November 2009.

[2] Nadine Fréry et al: EXPOSURE OF EMPLOYEES TO MULTIPLE CARCINOGENIC NUISANCES IN 2010. Soumis le 10.03.2017 // Date of submission: 03.10.2017

[3] RISK MONITORING AND PREVENTION NETWORK PROFESSIONALS IN PACA: Mechanics and bodywork, Motor vehicle maintenance. Prevention in action for the health of employees and companies. www.sante-securite-paca.org. ... . By sector

[4] CENTER NATIONAL DE LA RECHERCHE SCIENTIFIQUE :
Occupational risk assessment. Document unique Circulaire N° 6 DRT du 18 avril 2002. Implementing decree no. 2001-1016 creating a *risk* assessment *document.*

[5] EVENS EMMANUEL: Evaluation des risques sanitaires et éco toxicologiques lies aux effluents hospitaliers - Thèse de doctorat 2004.

[6] SYNERGIE ECOLE. COMPANY: Vehicle Maintenance Automobiles. Prevention in the Pays de la Loire region.

[7] SCTRICK L.: Evaluation des risques professionnels dans les établissements de santé. Hazard: intrinsic property or capacity of a piece of equipment.

[8] S A DIA et al: Assessment of occupational risks among workers at a flour mill in Dakar. https://www.sciencedirect.com/journal/archives-des-maladies-professionnelles-et-de-lenvironnement/vol/79/issue/1.   February 2018, Pages 18-22

[9] **S A DIA et al**: **S A DIA et al**: Assessment of occupational risks in the artisanal aluminum foundry sector in Dakar. https://www.sciencedirect.com/journal/archives-des-maladies-professionnelles-et-de-lenvironnement. October 2017, Pages 454-459

[10] **MATCHUM KOUOGUE CHRISTELLE F.-A.:** La protection juridique de l'environnement au Cameroun et en France le cas des nuisances sonores. University of Limoges - Master 2 thesis in International and Comparative Environmental Law 2008.

[11] **B Y Yeboué et al**: **B Y Yeboué et al**: Assessment of noise risk at 881 workstations in 320 private sector companies in Côte d'Ivoire. https://www.sciencedirect.com/journal/archives-des-maladies-professionnelles-et-de-lenvironnement/vol/79/issue/4. September 2018, Pages 528-533

[12] *INRS*: Evaluation des Risques professionnels. Aide au repérage des risques dans les PME - PMI. March 2011. www.travail-emploi.guov.fr, "Santé au Travail" tab.

[13] **CATHEL KORNIG AND ÉRIC VERDIER**: De très petites entreprises de la réparation automobile face aux normes publiques de la prévention des risques professionnels. Le cas d'une action collective territoriale. http://www.lest.cnrs.fr/IMG/pdf/Kornig_Verdier_RFAS.pdf

[14] *INRS*: Evaluation des Risques professionnels. Aide au repérage des risques dans les PME - PMI. March 2011. www.travail-emploi.guov.fr, Onglet " Santé au Travail ".

KNOWLEDGE, STUDIES AND PRACTICES OF NURSING STAFF AT THE CENTER NATIONAL D'APPAREILLAGE ORTHOPEDIQUE DU MALI IN THE FACE OF COVID 19

I Sacko[1] , H Kinta[2] , A Kiré[3] , A Samaké[4] , TB Bagayoko[5,] S Sanogo[6] , L Diakité[7] , FB TOURE[8] , B Diallo[9] , B Gakou[10,] (SOMASST) [11]

15. Mali National Orthopedic Fitting Center

16. Mali National Orthopedic Fitting Center

17. Mali National Orthopedic Fitting Center

18. Mali National Orthopedic Fitting Center

19. Forensic and occupational medicine department at the Nianankoro Fomba hospital in Ségou.

20. Agence Nationale d'Assistance Médicale (Bamako Mali)

21. Pelengana Sud Community Health Center (Ségou Mali)

22. Institut National de Prévoyance Sociale (Mali)

23. Caisse Malienne de Sécurité Sociale (Mali)

24. Cabinet Médical KENEYA (Bamako Mali).

25. Société Malienne de Santé Sécurité au Travail

Author: Dr Idrissa Sacko, Occupational Health and Safety Specialist, Centre National d'Appareillage Orthopédique. 00223 76 18 88 82

Email : sackoidrissa43@yahoo.fr

Conflict of interest: none

Summary:

Introduction: healthcare workers in particular, those who come into contact with patients or provide them with care, are more likely to be infected with SARS-CoV-2 than the general population.

Aim: The aim of our work was to study the knowledge, attitudes and practices of nursing staff at the Centre National d'Appareillage Orthopédique du Mali with regard to Covid-19.

Methodology: This was a descriptive cross-sectional study running from 1er to June 30 2020. It involved all CNAOM staff. The data collected were processed using SPSS (version 20.0) and EXCEL (version 17) software, and the texts were processed using Microsoft Word. Results: The participation rate was 100%, with an average age of 40.25 years and extremes ranging from 20 to 60 years. Our sample consisted of 07 women (15.9%) and 37 men (84.1%), with a clear male predominance, with a sex ratio of 5.28% in favor of men. Television was the most cited source of information in our study with 65.9%, in contrast to broadcasting with 31.8%. In our study, 97.7% of nursing staff believed in the existence of the pandemic. Several modes of transmission were mentioned, with respiratory droplets emphasized in 47.7% of cases. The majority of participants had a good knowledge of the clinical signs of the disease. In our study, the preferred attitude of nursing staff was to avoid physical contact with patients. In our study, 90.9% of staff had physical contact with patients, compared with 9.1%. In our study, barrier measures were not respected by patients (31.8%). The risk of exposure to disease was very high at

63.6%. Concerning stress, 72.7% of staff stated that the degree of stress was very high. As means of protection, the wearing of masks was the most common at 81.8%, followed by the use of hydroalcoholic gel at 9.1. In our study, 94.6% of nursing staff were satisfied with the implementation of the pandemic crisis committee. **Conclusion**: This serious and deadly pandemic deserves special attention.

Key words: Knowledge; Attitudes; Practices; Nursing staff; COVID-19; CNAOM

INTRODUCTION

The World Health Organization (WHO) has received an alert about a case of atypical pneumonia that appeared in Wuhan (China) on December 31, 2019 [5].

Investigations revealed that a new coronavirus was circulating, causing what we now know as "coronavirus disease 2019" (COVID-19).

On March 11, 2020, the epidemic of novel coronavirus disease was officially declared a pandemic by the WHO after having been declared a public health emergency of international concern on January 30, 2020. [6, 7]

In Africa, the epidemiological situation as of June 12, 2020, according to the African Union's Center for Disease Prevention and Control, the pandemic has reported 216,446 confirmed cases and 5,756 deaths on the continent [8]. The Maghreb countries were the first to be affected, notably Egypt, which was one of the first countries to report imported cases, Algeria and Morocco [8].

The first cases of the Covid-19 pandemic were recorded in Mali from March 25, 2020[10]. An official press release announced that two Malians had returned from France on March 12 and 16 respectively.

The first is a 49-year-old woman living in Bamako and the second a 62-year-old man living in Kayes (west of the country). According to a government press release dated June 10, 2020, the pandemic has reported 1,667 contaminated cases, 96 deaths and

948 cured cases [9]. With a view to contributing to better prevention of this pandemic, we felt it necessary to carry out this study on the knowledge, attitudes and practices of nursing staff at the Centre National d'Appareillage Orthopédique du Mali (CNAO) in relation to Covid-19.

I-MATERIALS AND METHOD

1.1- Study setting: The study was carried out at the Centre National d'Appareillage Orthopédique du Mali (CNAOM).

1.2- Type and period of study: This was a descriptive cross-sectional study from June 1 to June 30, 2020.

1.3- Study population: The study involved all nursing staff at the Centre National d'Appareillage Orthopédique in Mali.

1.4- Sampling: All nursing staff were included in the study.

1.5- Inclusion criteria: All nursing staff were included in our study.

1.6- Non-inclusion criteria: Administrative staff who had no direct contact with patients.

1.7- Data collection techniques and tools: Participants were asked to complete an anonymous individual questionnaire. In addition to socio-demographic and occupational data, the questionnaire included an assessment of participants' knowledge and attitudes towards coronavirus disease. The data collected were processed using SPSS (version 20.0) and EXCEL (version 17) software, and text processing was carried out using Microsoft Word.

II. RESULTS

1- Socio-demographic characteristics of participants

Table I: Age distribution.

Age	Workforce	Percentage
20 to 30 years	7	15,9
31 to 40 years	27	61,4
41 to 50 years	7	15,9
51 to 60 years	3	6,8
Total	44	100,0

Table II: Breakdown by gender.

Gender	Workforce	Percentage
Men	37	84,1

Woman	7	15,9
Total	44	100,0

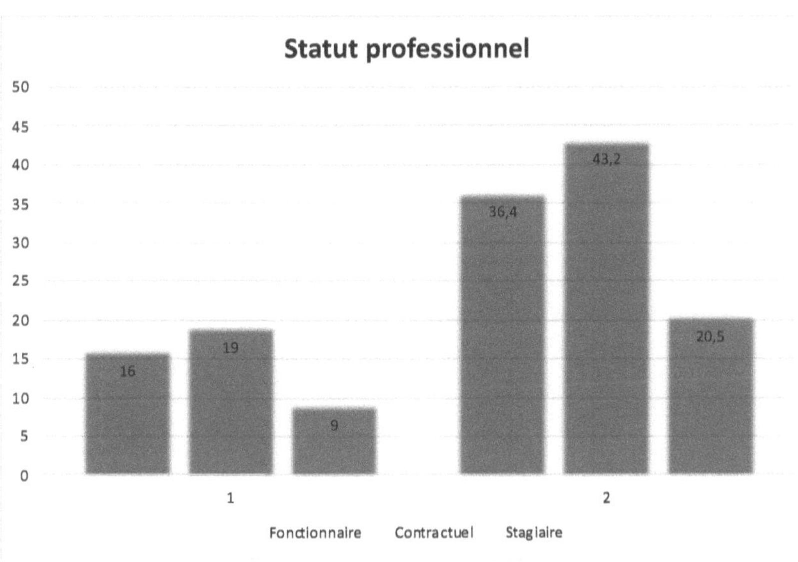

Figure 1: Distribution by professional status.

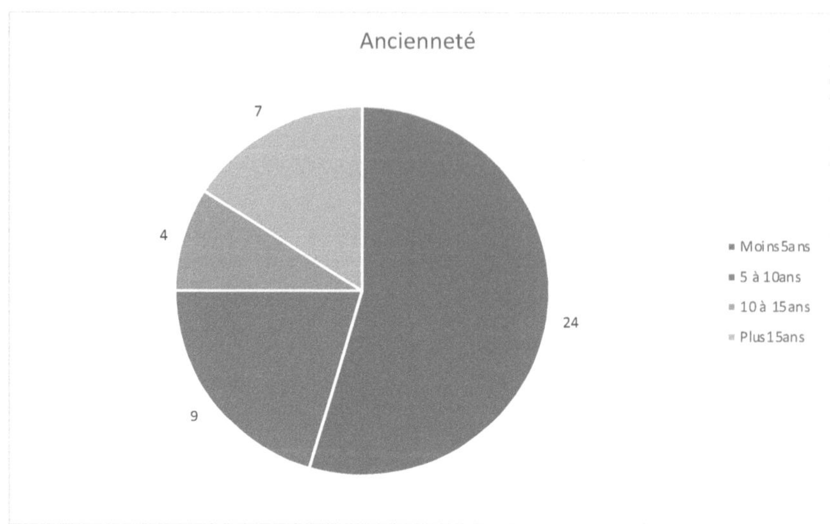

Figure 2: Breakdown by seniority.

2-Participants' knowledge of the disease

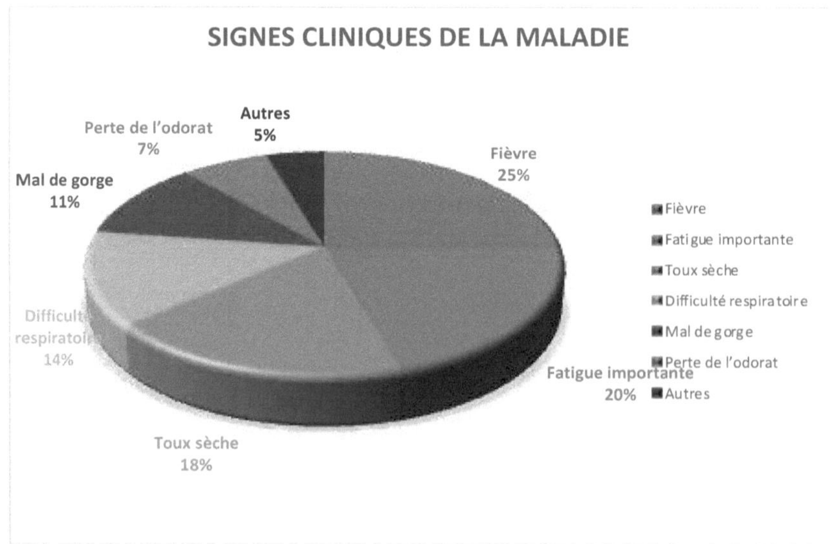

Figure 3: Knowledge by clinical signs of the disease

Table III: Distribution according to knowledge of mode of transmission

Distribution by transmission mode

mode of transmission	Workforce	Percentage
Respiratory droplets	21	47,7
Close contacts	20	45,4
Other	3	6,9
Total	44	100,0

3-Prevention practices

Table IV: Distribution according to knowledge of means of protection.

Means of protection	Workforce	Percentage
Mask	36	81,8
Glove	2	4,5

Hydroalcoholic gel	4	9,1
Distancing	2	4,5
Total	44	100,0

Table V: Satisfaction with the creation of a Covid -19 crisis committee.

Reaction of satisfaction	Workforce	Percentage
Satisfied	42	95,4
Not satisfied	2	4,6
Total	44	100,0

The participation rate in our study was 100%. The most represented group was 61.4%. This result is lower than that of L DIAKITE in 58.1% of cases [1]. In our study, males accounted for 84.1%. The low proportion of women in our sample can be explained by the fact that few women work in these professions. In the Mamadou Maktar Mbacké Leye study, 66.5% were male [4]. In our study, INFSS students were the most represented in our sample, with 20.5%. In contrast, in M SANOGO's study, the most represented category was general practitioners with 30.2% [3]. The reason for this difference is that students in training were the most numerous to participate in our study.

 Knowledge of the pandemic: In our study, television was the most cited source of information, with 65.9%. This compares with 31.8% for radio broadcasting. This result is comparable to that of L DIAKITE et Al [1].

Belief in the existence of the disease: In 97.7% of cases, nursing staff believed in the existence of the pandemic. This result is comparable to that of Mamadou Makhtar Mbacké Leye, who found 94.8% [4].

Mode of transmission: Several modes of transmission were mentioned, with 47.7% of participants emphasizing respiratory droplets and 45.4% close contact. This result is lower than that of M. SANOGO, who found 63% for respiratory droplets [3]. Clinical signs: In our study, the majority of participants had a good knowledge of clinical signs.

The possibility of recovery: In our study, 52.2% of people said that an infected person could recover. This result is lower than that of M SANOGO, who found 63% [3].

Attitude to the pandemic: In our study, the preferred attitude of care staff was to avoid physical contact with patients. In our study, 90.9% of care staff had physical contact with patients, compared with 9.1%.

In our study, barrier measures were not respected by patients (31.8%). Risk of exposure to the disease: In our study, the risk of exposure to the disease was very high, at 63.6%. This result is comparable to that of the study by L DIAKITE et Al, which found a very high risk of exposure to the disease [1]. Degree of stress: 72.7% of operatives stated that the degree of stress was very high, compared with 28.9% in the L DIAKITE et Al study [1]. Means of protection: Masks were the most common means of protection, with 81.8%, followed by the use of hydroalcoholic gel (9.1%). In Mamadou Makhtar Mbacké Leye's study, 93.8% wore masks, and 77.8% washed their hands with soap and water [4]. Regular replacement of protective equipment 65.9% of staff confirmed regular replacement of protective equipment. Room hygiene was 56.8% according to participants. Satisfaction of nursing staff with the setting up of the crisis committee and management of Covid-19. The aim of the crisis committee was to describe the preventive measures put in place by our health authorities, but also to develop our own barrier measures and adapt them to our working environment to ensure staff protection against the pandemic. In our study, 94.6% of nursing staff had a positive reaction to the setting up of the pandemic crisis committee. This was also the case in the M KONE study [2]. Staff suggestions for improving pandemic prevention: 63.6% of nursing staff recommended reducing the number of patients at the entrance, while 31.8% were in favor of reducing the number of staff in the room. According to the degree of satisfaction by workstation, 54.5% of staff found the measures insufficient. The reinforcement of preventive measures to improve prevention against the pandemic, the same recommendation was found in the study by Lamine Diakité [1].

IV. BIBLIOGRAPHICAL REFERENCES

1. L DIAKITE et Al. Knowledge, attitudes and practices of healthcare professionals regarding Covid-19 infection in Mali.

2. M KONE .What strategies to protect workers against Covid-19 in a mining sector in Mali?

3. M SANOGO. Évaluation des pratiques d'hygiène et de prévention de la maladie à coronavirus en milieu hospitalier : Cas des centers d'isolement et de traitement du covid19 au Centre Hospitalo-Universitaire du Point G (CHU-PG) au Mali.

4. Mamadou Makhtar Mbacké Leye. Knowledge, attitudes and practices of the population of the Dakar region regarding COVID-19.

5. World Health Organization (2020) - Pneumonia of unknown cause - China, available at <https://https://www.who.int/csr/don/05-january-2020-pneumonia-of-unkown-cause-china/fr/>. Accessed April 30, 2020

6. World Health Organization (2020) - Statement on the second meeting of the Emergency Committee of the International Health Regulations (2005) concerning the outbreak of new coronavirus 2019 (2019-nCoV), available at <https://www.who.int/fr/news-room/detail/30-01-2020-statement-on-the-second-meeting-of-the-international-health-regulations-(2005)-emergency-committee-regarding-the-outbreak-of-novel-coronavirus-(2019-ncov) >. Accessed April 30, 2020

7. World Health Organization (2020) - Keynote address by the WHO Director-General at the press briefing on COVID-19: March 11, 2020, available at < https://www.who.int/fr/dg/speeches/detail/who-director-general-s-opening-remarks-at-the-media-briefing-on-covid-19---11-march-2020>. Accessed April 30, 2020

8. Arica CDC: African Centers for Disease Control and Prevention.

9. Communicating with the Ministry of Health and **Social** Affairs

TABLE OF CONTENTS

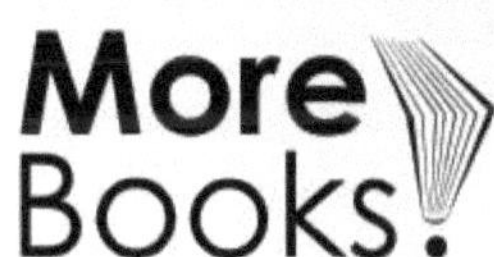

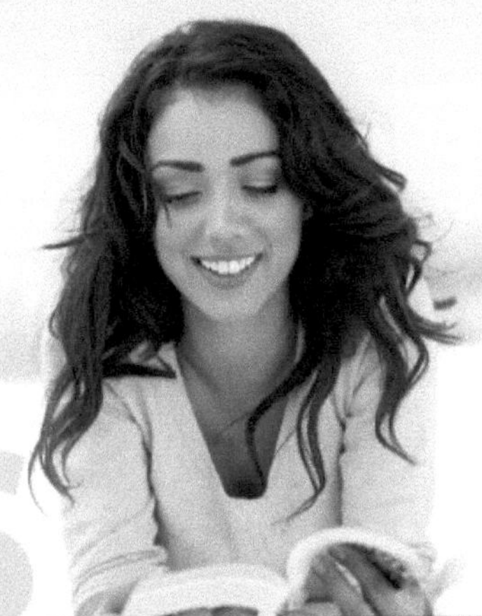

yes I want morebooks!

Buy your books fast and straightforward online - at one of world's fastest growing online book stores! Environmentally sound due to Print-on-Demand technologies.

Buy your books online at
www.morebooks.shop

Kaufen Sie Ihre Bücher schnell und unkompliziert online – auf einer der am schnellsten wachsenden Buchhandelsplattformen weltweit! Dank Print-On-Demand umwelt- und ressourcenschonend produziert.

Bücher schneller online kaufen
www.morebooks.shop

info@omniscriptum.com
www.omniscriptum.com

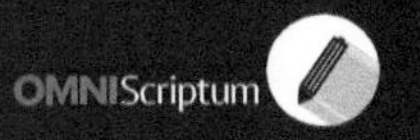

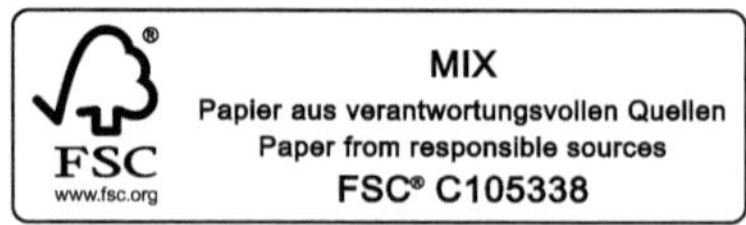
MIX
Papier aus verantwortungsvollen Quellen
Paper from responsible sources
FSC® C105338
FSC
www.fsc.org